From Unknown Addiction to Intentional Achievement

A Unique System to Eradicate Drugs, Alcohol and Negative Addictions

By

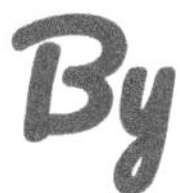

Samuel C.A Adolphus

3

Introduction

The Vision Behind This Book;

This book is a helpful and life changing book, aimed at educating people who are victims of drugs, alcohol and any other negative kind of addiction. This book is created to actually charge the urge for a positive life and to educate and help eradicate any kind of negative addiction in individuals.

A New Path for Lasting Recovery; Acknowledging the scale of the drug and alcohol addiction crisis, both on a personal and societal level, this book teaches the traditional methods of addiction recovery.

This book is helpful for every victim of addiction, providing long-term solutions. It highlight's and inspires with the development of a unique system to cure addiction. Not only for people who tackle addiction but also empowers individuals to live fulfilling, and meaningful lives.

Personal Motivation and Expertise: From my life experiences, I've seen lots of harm, mayhem, and havoc caused by drugs, alcohol, sex and even gambling addicts. I've been a victim of the effects caused by these addicts in society. I have come up with a solution in this book for my readers, individuals and everyone who is looking for guidance. You all need to know that I'm the right person to provide it. This book involves my personal battle with addiction, my experience as a recovery counselor, and my extensive research in the field.

Empowering Change: This book also outline's the idea that recovery is more than just quitting drugs or alcohol. True recovery involves rebuilding one's life, achieving self-empowerment, and discovering a deeper sense of purpose. This book is a full guide to not only help individuals overcome addiction but also lead them toward personal achievement and success.

Why This Approach Is Different; This book creates a unique system from the common methods of addiction treatment and recovery.

Holistic, Comprehensive Approach: This book also explains that, this book isn't just about quitting an addiction, but it's about building a new life. Where many traditional approaches focus solely on abstinence, your system integrates the physical, emotional, and mental aspects of recovery. This book details how this method promotes healing on multiple levels: physical detoxification, emotional resilience, mental clarity, and spiritual well-being tailored to Individual Needs: Many recovery programs take a one-size-fits-all approach, but addiction is a deeply personal struggle. The book describes how your system offers flexibility and can be adapted to each individual's unique situation, personality, and pace of recovery. This book explains how this adaptability enhances its effectiveness, allowing people to make meaningful, lasting changes in their lives.

Long-Term, Sustainable Change: The goal isn't just sobriety but long-term transformation. The book discusses how this system encourages individuals to build habits, mindsets, and routines that will keep them not only free from addiction but thriving in other areas of life. Highlight that the approach fosters self-responsibility and growth beyond addiction recovery, aiming to help individuals achieve their full potential.

How to Use This Book Effectively

This book will guide readers and individuals on how to eradicate addiction and gradually exhibit a better life, and have the mindset, mentality and ability of achievement. So,

1. Follow the Journey Step by Step.

2. I'm encouraging all my readers and individuals to view the book as a roadmap rather than a quick fix.

3. Each chapter builds upon the previous one, guiding them through the stages of recovery, from understanding your addiction to achieving long-term fulfillment. I advise readers to approach each section with patience, allowing time for reflection and personal growth.

About The Author

Samuel C.A Adolphus is a high-performance psychologist recognized for his work(s) in helping individuals and teams excel in high-stakes environments.
He is also a very professional musician, singer, multi-instrumentalist, songwriter and dancer.
His expertise has been sought by High classed business men, 16 other companies, NFL teams, government and non-governmental organizations.

Table Of Contents

<u>Summary</u>

<u>Acknowledgments</u>

<u>References</u>

Chapter 1: Defining Drugs and Alcohol Addiction

Understanding Addiction: A Comprehensive Look at Substance Dependence

Addiction is often seen in a simplistic light, frequently misunderstood as merely a matter of weak willpower. However, it's a profound and chronic condition that influences every aspect of a person's existence. This exploration aims to shed light on addiction as much more than just drug or alcohol use.

Picture addiction as a dominating force. It's not a mere habit but rather resembles a disease that changes how the brain functions and influences decision-making and behavior. Addiction involves compulsive substance use despite adverse consequences, much like how no one would opt for an illness such as cancer or diabetes.

Addiction affects both body and mind. Visualize the internal struggle of someone caught in its grip. Physically, their body becomes reliant on the substance to feel normal, while mentally, they endure intense cravings and emotional distress that make quitting seem impossible.

Consider the brain's reward system as a traffic signal. Substances trigger the green light, urging "go, feel good!" due to a surge in dopamine. But addiction breaks this signal. The brain continuously chases that green light, overlooking dangers like health issues or strained relationships. With ongoing use, the body adjusts, needing more of the substance to achieve the same high, a concept known as tolerance, leading to withdrawal when the substance isn't used.

Tolerance means the body requires greater amounts of the substance for the same effect, and withdrawal makes stopping punishingly difficult. Withdrawal can bring severe anxiety, tremors, nausea, and even seizures, making quitting not only tough but physically and emotionally tormenting.

Psychologically, triggers and cravings act like invisible chains, binding a person to their habit. Everyday occurrences like walking past a bar, hearing a specific song, or feeling stress can ignite a powerful urge to use again. These cravings are deeply rooted in the brain's chemistry.

Exploring the Brain's Role in Addiction

Delving into the brain helps us understand addiction from a biological standpoint. The brain acts as a control center and starts malfunctioning under the influence of drugs or alcohol. Substance use increases dopamine, a neurotransmitter linked to pleasure. Normally, dopamine is released during enjoyable activities like eating or spending time with loved ones. However, substances release much higher levels, overwhelming the brain.

Continuous substance use rewires the brain. It begins prioritizing drugs or alcohol over natural rewards such as relationships or responsibilities, fixating on obtaining the next fix. Over time, brain circuits related to reward, stress, and self-control become so altered that rational decisions about substance use become impossible. At this stage, the choice to use is overshadowed by the brain's demands.

Addiction also impairs the brain's response to negative consequences. Even when aware of the harm caused, the brain seeks relief through more substance use, perpetuating the addiction cycle.

The Promise of Neuroplasticity

The brain's capacity to adapt, known as neuroplasticity, offers hope. Recovery can rewire the brain, reversing damage and restoring healthier thought and behavior patterns. This journey is more than overcoming physical dependence; it's about retraining the brain to find pleasure in healthy ways.

Lingering Effects on Brain Function

Even after substance use stops, addiction leaves lasting marks on the brain. Many in recovery struggle with impaired memory, decision-making, and emotional regulation.

Imagine trying to navigate life with a foggy mind, unpredictable emotions, and difficulty concentrating. Recovery goes beyond detox; it's about healing the brain, requiring time, patience, and support. While the brain's ability to repair is remarkable, recovery, like addiction, is a gradual process.

Chapter 2: Understanding the Roots of Addiction: *Triggers, Causes, and Risk Factors*

In this chapter, we explore the complex web of factors leading to addiction, shedding light on why some individuals are more prone to substance abuse. By delving into the psychological, environmental, and genetic components at play, readers will gain a thorough understanding of how addiction begins and why overcoming it requires addressing more than just the physical dependency. This examination includes the emotional distress and trauma often behind addictive behaviors, as well as the societal and cultural forces that maintain patterns of substance misuse.

This section will cover several pivotal areas, these areas are as follows:

- Understanding Addiction: Beyond Just Substance Dependency
- Emotional and Psychological Triggers: The Role of Trauma and Mental Health
- Environmental and Social Influences: The Context of Addiction
- Genetic Factors: The Hereditary Elements of Addiction
- Co-occurring Disorders: The Link Between Addiction and Mental Health
- Cultural and Societal Influences on Addiction
- Stress and Coping Mechanisms in Addiction
- Viewing Addiction as a Disease: The Limits of Willpower
- The Impact of Early Life Experiences on Addiction Risk
- Breaking the Cycle: Addressing Root Causes in Recovery

1. Understanding Addiction: Beyond Just Substance Dependency

We begin by challenging the notion that addiction is purely about the substance itself. It's a common misconception that drugs and alcohol's chemical properties are the only causes, but the reality is much more intricate. Substances like heroin, marijuana, cocaine, and alcohol can create physical dependency by altering the brain's reward systems, yet addiction often starts well before the first use.

Many who struggle with addiction resort to substances to cope with deeper emotional, psychological, or social issues. For instance, one might drink to deal with loneliness or use drugs to escape trauma or depression. These underlying emotional drivers mean that even after detoxifying from the physical dependency, the addiction can persist if these foundational issues remain unaddressed. It's not just the addictive substance but the unresolved emotional pain that compels individuals to return to it.

2. Emotional and Psychological Triggers: The Role of Trauma and Mental Health

This segment delves into the emotional and psychological aspects making individuals more susceptible to addiction. Trauma, depression, anxiety, and other forms of emotional distress are significant triggers for substance use. Many battling addiction essentially self-medicate, using drugs or alcohol to dull their emotional pain.

Individuals who've experienced major traumas, such as childhood abuse or a loved one's loss, might feel emotionally overwhelmed and turn to substances for short-term relief. These substances provide a temporary escape but create a strong psychological dependence as the brain begins to associate substance use with emotional pain relief. Mental health disorders like depression, anxiety, PTSD, and bipolar disorder frequently accompany addiction. Without appropriate treatment, substance use can worsen mental health issues, creating a vicious cycle.

3. Environmental and Social Influences: The Context of Addiction

This section highlights the significant role of one's environment and social settings in shaping addiction. Factors such as family dynamics, peer influence, socioeconomic status, and cultural norms greatly impact addiction risk. For instance, individuals growing up in environments where substance use is normalized or where emotional support is missing are at higher risk.

During adolescence, peer pressure is particularly influential. Teens who hang out with peers who use drugs or alcohol are more likely to adopt these behaviors. Environmental stressors like poverty, unemployment, or exposure to violence can also significantly contribute to addiction, as individuals might turn to substances for escape.

Recognizing how these factors interact underscores why altering one's environment or support network can be crucial for recovery.

4. Genetic Factors: The Hereditary Elements of Addiction

Exploring genetic influences reveals that while addiction isn't solely determined by genetics, there is a substantial hereditary component. Some people might inherit traits making their brains more sensitive to drugs or alcohol, thus increasing their addiction risk.

Research indicates that addiction often runs in families. If a close relative has struggled with substance abuse, a person is more likely to face similar challenges due to genetic factors and the environment of growing up around substance use. Although a genetic predisposition doesn't seal one's fate, it emphasizes the need for awareness and preventive measures against substance misuse.

5. Co-occurring Disorders: The Link Between Addiction and Mental Health

Addiction frequently coexists with mental health issues like anxiety, depression, or PTSD, making treatment more complicated. For example, someone with anxiety might use alcohol to calm their nerves temporarily, but since alcohol is a depressant, it eventually exacerbates their anxiety, creating a harmful cycle.

Effective treatment must address both the mental health disorder and the addiction simultaneously. Integrated treatment plans involving therapy, medication, and support groups can help individuals manage both their mental health and substance use more effectively.

6. Cultural and Societal Influences on Addiction

This section examines how cultural norms and societal pressures impact addiction. In many cultures, substance use is either glamorized or expected in certain settings, making it difficult for individuals to recognize when their use has become problematic. Societal pressures to excel in work or academics might drive individuals towards substances promising temporary relief or enhanced performance.

Certain subcultures, such as nightlife or high-stress industries, foster environments where substance use is prevalent. Additionally, societal stigma and judgment regarding addiction can prevent individuals from seeking help, highlighting the need for cultural changes to support recovery efforts.

7. Stress and Coping Mechanisms in Addiction

Stress is a common trigger for substance use, especially when individuals lack healthy coping mechanisms. While stress is a part of everyday life, the way we handle it greatly influences whether we turn to substances. Those lacking healthy outlets, like exercise, meditation, or therapy, are more likely to use drugs or alcohol to cope, adding more issues to their lives.

This section underscores the importance of developing healthy coping strategies as a key element of the recovery process.

8. Viewing Addiction as a Disease: The Limits of Willpower

This part clarifies that overcoming addiction isn't just a matter of willpower. Addiction is a disease affecting brain function, particularly in areas responsible for pleasure, reward, and decision-making. Just as chronic illnesses like diabetes require medical treatment and lifestyle adjustments, so does addiction.

Recognizing that addiction involves changes in brain function highlights why professional treatment and support are crucial, and why sheer willpower isn't enough for sustained recovery.

9. The Impact of Early Life Experiences on Addiction Risk

Early life experiences play a significant role in addiction risk. Adverse childhood experiences (ACEs) like abuse, neglect, or growing up in unstable environments are strong predictors of future substance abuse. Trauma during formative years can have long-lasting effects on emotional and psychological health.

Children from unstable environments often develop coping mechanisms to manage their pain, which may later manifest as substance use. Discussing factors like attachment theory, intergenerational trauma, and early stress's impact on brain development helps illustrate these connections.

Resilience factors, such as strong social support and positive role models, can mitigate these risks, highlighting that while early experiences shape vulnerability, they don't determine an individual's destiny.

10. Breaking the Cycle: Addressing Root Causes in Recovery

In this concluding section, we stress the importance of addressing the fundamental causes of addiction for successful recovery. Recovery isn't just about abstaining from substance use; it requires healing underlying emotional, psychological, and social issues. An effective recovery plan examines emotional triggers, coping mechanisms, and unresolved traumas.

Therapy, particularly trauma-informed therapy, can help individuals process past experiences and develop healthier coping techniques. Building a supportive network is crucial, whether through support groups, sober living communities, or friendships.

Ultimately, addiction is a complex and challenging condition, but addressing its root causes makes recovery attainable. Viewing addiction as a coping mechanism for deeper, unresolved pain shifts the focus from blame to compassionate treatment. This chapter sets the tone for the rest of the book, leading readers to address these core issues and work towards a healthier, substance-free life.

Chapter 3: The Stages of Addiction and Recovery: *Recognizing the Cycle and the Path to Freedom*

In this chapter, we take an in-depth look at the stages of addiction and the journey toward recovery. Addiction is a gradual process, starting from initial experimentation and potentially leading to full dependency. Similarly, the recovery journey also unfolds through multiple phases, involving both healing and personal growth. By understanding these stages, individuals can more precisely identify where they stand in the cycle and the steps necessary for progress. This chapter aims to guide you through the complexities of addiction and recovery, helping to recognize addictive behaviors while offering a hopeful roadmap for achieving lasting freedom and sobriety.

Here are the key topics we'll examine:

- The Gradual Nature of Addiction: From Initial Experimentation to Full Dependency
- Unpacking Addiction: Physical, Emotional, and Mental Dependence
- Denial and Justification: The Addict's Mental Defense
- The Turning Point: Recognizing the Shift from Use to Abuse
- The Challenge of Withdrawal: Physical and Psychological Symptoms
- The Path to Recovery: Transitioning from Survival to Thriving
- Precontemplation: Unrecognized Problem
- Contemplation: Acknowledging the Need for Change
- Preparation: Planning and Taking Initial Steps to Quit
- Action: Implementing Steps Toward Recovery

1. The Gradual Nature of Addiction: From Initial Experimentation to Full Dependency

Addiction develops over time, starting with casual or experimental use that seems harmless. Many people begin using substances out of curiosity, due to peer pressure, or to cope with stress, often convinced they are in control and that occasional use won't lead to problems. However, as time passes, this occasional use can become more frequent. The brain starts to build a tolerance, requiring more of the substance to achieve the same effect, leading to dependency.

2. Unpacking Addiction: Physical, Emotional, and Mental Dependence

To fully understand addiction, it's essential to look at it through three lenses: physical, emotional, and mental. Addiction is not just about physical cravings; it also involves emotional and psychological components.

- <u>Physical Dependence;</u> occurs when the body adapts to the substance and experiences withdrawal symptoms if the substance is removed.

- <u>Emotional Dependence;</u> involves using the substance as a mechanism to cope with feelings such as stress, sadness, or fear, making the individual feel incapable of handling their emotions without it.

- <u>Mental Dependence is</u> characterized by an obsessive focus on the substance, manifesting in cravings and compulsive behavior.

By examining these dimensions, we can see how addiction impacts not just the body but also the mind and emotions.

3. Denial and Justification: The Addict's Mental Defense

Denial is a powerful obstacle in overcoming addiction. Many individuals convince themselves their substance use isn't a problem. They may believe they can quit anytime, that their use isn't harming their life, or that they need the substance to function.

Justification occurs when people find excuses to rationalize their substance use, such as "I've had a tough day," "I deserve to unwind," or "Everyone else is doing it." These mental defenses prevent them from confronting the true impact of their behavior.

Understanding these mental tricks can help individuals break through denial and justification, encouraging an honest assessment of their substance use and its consequences.

4. The Turning Point: Recognizing the Shift from Use to Abuse

A critical moment in the addiction journey is when substance use transitions from being occasional to becoming abusive. This shift can be gradual or sudden but is crucial to identify.

This turning point often happens when substance use starts to overshadow responsibilities like work, relationships, or health. The substance goes from being an occasional pleasure to a necessity for feeling normal.

5. The Challenge of Withdrawal: Physical and Psychological Symptoms

The fear of withdrawal often keeps people trapped in addiction. This section explains the symptoms of withdrawal based on the type of substance and why they occur.

Withdrawal symptoms can range from mild, like headaches and nausea, to severe, like seizures and hallucinations. Knowing what to expect during withdrawal and learning how to manage these symptoms is crucial. Though difficult, withdrawal is a temporary phase on the road to long-term recovery.

6. The Path to Recovery: Transitioning from Survival to Thriving

Recovery is a gradual process, unfolding in stages just like addiction. It's important for those in recovery to understand that healing takes time and that setbacks are part of the journey.

The stages include:

- <u>Precontemplation</u>: Not yet acknowledging the problem.
- <u>Contemplation</u>: Recognizing the issue and considering change.

- <u>Preparation</u>: Planning and taking initial steps toward change.
- <u>Action</u>: Implementing steps such as joining a treatment program.
- <u>Maintenance</u>: Working to sustain recovery and avoid relapse.
- <u>Relapse</u>: Learning from setbacks and recommitting to the recovery plan.
- <u>Long-term Recovery</u>: Embracing a sober life and continuing personal growth.

This section will provide details on each stage, helping individuals understand their journey and what to expect.

7. <u>Precontemplation</u>: Unrecognized Problem

In the precontemplation stage, individuals haven't yet admitted they have an addiction. They might deny the problem, thinking their substance use is under control or not affecting their lives negatively.

8. <u>Contemplation</u>: Acknowledging the Need for Change

During contemplation, individuals start to question their substance use and consider the possibility of change. This stage involves an internal struggle as they weigh the pros and cons of their substance use, recognizing its negative effects but fearing the changes recovery will bring.

9. <u>Preparation</u>: Planning and Taking Initial Steps to Quit

Once they acknowledge the need for change, individuals move into the preparation stage. They start making plans to quit by researching treatment options, speaking with counselors, or setting a quit date.

10. <u>Action</u>: Implementing Steps Toward Recovery

In the action stage, individuals take concrete steps to address their addiction. This might include entering detox or rehab programs, attending therapy, or joining support groups.

Early recovery can be emotionally intense, requiring strong support systems and coping strategies to manage cravings and the desire to use substances again. Essential steps in this stage include:

- Seeking Professional Help: Addiction is a medical condition that often requires professional intervention, such as detox, rehab, and therapy.
- Addressing Underlying Issues: Recovery involves dealing with the emotional and psychological issues that contribute to addiction.
- Building New Routines: Part of recovery is restructuring daily life to replace old habits with new, healthier routines like

exercising, practicing mindfulness, and developing new hobbies.

By fully committing to these steps, individuals can build a strong foundation for a sustainable, substance-free life.

Chapter 4: *Creating an Action Plan: Building a Sustainable Path to Sobriety.*

In this chapter, we'll explore the process of crafting a thorough and sustainable plan to ensure long-term sobriety. An effective plan isn't merely about quitting substance use; it's about making significant lifestyle adjustments to support recovery. By this stage, individuals will have gained an understanding of addiction, its effects, and the necessity of recognizing the recovery stages. Now, the attention shifts to practical steps and actionable strategies to build a life free from addiction.

Formulating a robust action plan involves introspection, thoughtful planning, and commitment. It includes setting goals, identifying personal strengths and weaknesses, and developing strategies to overcome obstacles that may arise during recovery. This chapter will guide individuals through each step of this process, equipping them with the tools needed to create a personalized path toward lasting sobriety and a healthier lifestyle.

We will cover the following points in this chapter:

1. <u>Understanding the Importance of an Action Plan</u>
2. <u>Self-Assessment</u>: Knowing Your Strengths, Weaknesses, and Triggers
3. <u>Setting SMART Goals for Recovery</u>

1. Understanding the Importance of an Action Plan

We'll begin by explaining why it's essential to have an action plan for achieving and maintaining sobriety. Without a clear and structured plan, the recovery journey can feel daunting and aimless, making it easier to revert to old habits. An action plan provides direction, guiding individuals through daily decision-making and offering strategies for handling obstacles.

While quitting substances might seem like the ultimate goal, maintaining sobriety is the real challenge. To do this effectively, individuals need a roadmap that helps them navigate their day-to-day lives.

Additionally, an action plan helps keep individuals accountable. By committing to specific goals and writing them down, people in recovery can track their progress and stay motivated. This plan is not just a tool for the present but serves as a guide for lifelong sobriety and personal growth.

2. Self-Assessment: Knowing Your Strengths, Weaknesses, and Triggers

Before developing an action plan, an honest self-assessment is crucial. Let's take a deep dive into understanding our strengths, weaknesses, and triggers related to substance use.

Strengths: These are personal qualities, skills, and resources that will assist in the recovery journey, such as resilience, determination, problem-solving skills, and the ability to seek help. Readers will be encouraged to reflect on past challenges they've overcome and how these strengths can be leveraged in their recovery.

Weaknesses: It's also important to confront areas of vulnerability, such as poor stress management, a tendency to isolate, or a lack of healthy coping mechanisms. Acknowledging these weaknesses isn't about judgment; it's about recognizing where additional support or effort may be required.

Triggers: Identifying the people, places, and situations that provoke cravings for substances is essential. Triggers can be external (like a specific environment) or internal (such as stress, anxiety, or boredom).

3. Setting SMART Goals for Recovery

Goals are the cornerstone of any effective action plan. However, vague or unrealistic goals can result in frustration and failure. This section introduces individuals to the SMART framework for goal-setting:

- Specific: Goals should be clear and precise. Instead of saying, "I want to stop using drugs," a specific goal would be, "I want to complete a 30-day detox program."
- Measurable: Goals should include criteria for tracking progress, such as, "I will attend three therapy sessions a week."
- Achievable: Goals must be realistic given the individual's circumstances. Setting impossible goals can lead to discouragement.

- <u>Relevant</u>: Goals should be directly related to the recovery process and the individual's desire to lead a sober, healthy life.
- <u>Time-bound</u>: Goals should have deadlines or time frames to create a sense of urgency and accountability.

By the end of this chapter, individuals will have a detailed, actionable plan to support their journey toward long-term sobriety.

Chapter 5: Building a Life of Achievement.

Breaking free from addiction is an incredible achievement, but it's just the beginning of a transformative journey. The real challenge lies in not only maintaining sobriety but also learning to lead a meaningful, fulfilling life afterward. This segment, "Building a Life of Achievement," aims to guide individuals through reclaiming their lives, setting achievable goals, and aiming for personal and professional excellence. This path involves crafting a balanced life, incorporating self-care into daily habits, and committing to ongoing personal growth.

Setting Personal, Professional, and Health Goals Post-Recovery

Transitioning from recovery to a life of achievement starts with setting clear, realistic goals. These goals act as a roadmap, directing individuals towards the future they aspire to. In post-recovery life, goal-setting should cover several key areas: personal development, professional ambitions, and physical health.

<u>Personal Goals</u>:
Post-recovery often brings a sense of rebirth. Personal goals might include mending relationships strained by addiction, exploring new hobbies, or building emotional resilience. Such goals help individuals rediscover their passions, boost self-esteem, and find a sense of purpose. Personal development can also involve engaging in therapeutic activities like journaling, mindfulness, or creative pursuits like art or music. These activities foster a sense of fulfillment and allow

individuals to explore their identities, which is crucial for long-term recovery.

<u>Professional Goals</u>:
Addiction frequently disrupts one's career, leaving a need to rebuild or start anew. Setting professional goals could involve returning to work, pursuing further education, or beginning a new business venture. It's essential to approach these goals with patience and persistence, acknowledging that rebuilding a successful career post-recovery takes time. Professional goals offer a sense of direction and accomplishment, leading to financial independence, self-confidence, and a sense of purpose, all vital for maintaining sobriety.

<u>Health Goals</u>:
Physical and mental health are foundational in recovery. Health goals might involve improving fitness, adopting a healthy diet, or addressing medical issues caused by

addiction. Recovery provides an opportunity to focus on restoring health. Regular exercise, proper nutrition, and mindfulness practices like meditation or yoga can help maintain a positive mindset and prevent relapse. Setting realistic health goals helps individuals build strength, improve mood, and enhance overall well-being.

When setting goals, it's important to ensure they are Smart, Specific, Measurable, Achievable, Relevant, and Time-bound. This structured approach helps individuals stay on track and measure their progress toward their objectives.

Creating a Balanced Life: Time Management and Self-Care

Living a fulfilling life post-recovery is about more than just reaching goals; it's about finding balance. Addiction often causes chaos, leading to a lack of structure.

Post-recovery life involves learning to manage time effectively and prioritize self-care.

Time Management:
During recovery, the importance of structure and routine becomes evident for maintaining stability. Effective time management is crucial for maintaining focus and reducing stress, which can help prevent relapse. Allocating time to personal, professional, and health goals without feeling overwhelmed is key.

Creating a Schedule:
An organized schedule serves as a daily roadmap. By allocating time for work, exercise, self-care, and relaxation, individuals can make progress towards their goals while also caring for their mental and physical well-being.

Prioritizing Tasks:

Not all tasks have equal importance. Learning to prioritize is a critical aspect of time management. Focusing on high-priority tasks first can reduce stress and boost productivity, helping individuals stay motivated and on track.

<u>Self-Care</u>:
Recovery is a long-term process, and prioritizing self-care is part of building a life of achievement. Self-care involves activities that nourish the body, mind, and spirit, allowing individuals to recharge and remain mentally and physically healthy.

- <u>Physical Self-Care</u>: Exercise, good nutrition, and adequate rest are vital for sustaining sobriety and fostering a sense of vitality. Physical self-care also regulates mood and energy levels, reducing emotional triggers that could lead to relapse.
- <u>Mental and Emotional Self-Care</u>: Emotional well-being is as important as

physical health. Mindfulness, therapy, and meditation help maintain emotional balance. Positive relationships and setting boundaries protect against stress and negative influences.

- <u>Social Self-Care</u>: Rebuilding social connections is essential. Surrounding oneself with supportive, positive people helps prevent feelings of isolation. Support groups, volunteering, or spending time with loved ones provide a sense of belonging.

Self-care is not a luxury but a necessity in post-recovery life. Incorporating it into daily routines ensures individuals stay resilient, balanced, and focused on their long-term goals.

Continuous Growth and Improvement

Achieving sobriety is a significant milestone, but it marks the beginning of a lifelong journey of self-improvement. Continuous growth is essential for maintaining a sense of purpose and avoiding complacency. Recovery is dynamic, with always room for further development, both personally and professionally.

Lifelong Learning:

Continuous growth involves a commitment to lifelong learning. Whether gaining new skills for career advancement, exploring personal interests, or learning more about addiction and recovery, ongoing education equips individuals with the tools to evolve and grow.

Personal Development:

Growth can take many forms, from improving communication skills to learning stress management. Focusing on personal development enhances emotional intelligence, strengthens relationships, and improves overall quality of life.

Professional Development:

Career growth is part of achieving long-term success. This could involve pursuing certifications, attending workshops, or networking. Staying engaged with career goals maintains focus and motivation, preventing a sense of stagnation that can sometimes lead to relapse.

Embracing New Challenges:
Continued growth means stepping out of comfort zones and embracing new challenges. This might mean pursuing a new career, learning a new skill, or setting ambitious personal goals. Facing challenges with determination and resilience builds self-confidence and reinforces that recovery is not just about survival but thriving.

Maintaining a Supportive Environment:
Growth requires a strong support system. Whether through peer support groups, therapy, or friendships, positive influences help individuals stay committed to recovery and personal growth.

<u>Celebrating Achievements</u>:
It's important to celebrate achievements, no matter how small. Recognizing milestones in recovery and personal development fosters a sense of accomplishment and reinforces the value of continuous growth. Every achievement, from professional goals to maintaining a health routine or staying sober for another day, deserves acknowledgment.

Conclusion

"Building a Life of Achievement" is about more than setting goals; it's about creating a balanced life that fosters continuous personal growth and fulfillment. By setting realistic personal, professional, and health goals, individuals in recovery can rebuild their lives. Effective time management and self-care are crucial for maintaining balance and staying on track. Through lifelong learning, embracing new challenges, and fostering a growth mindset, individuals can continue to evolve and thrive long after recovery.

Chapter 6: Turning Your Journey into Empowerment

One of the most profound benefits of recovery is the capacity to turn your personal challenges into a wellspring of strength and encouragement for others. This chapter shifts its attention from individual healing to the broader impact that your journey can have on those facing similar struggles. By sharing your story, offering support, and advocating for change, you can transform the difficulties of addiction into opportunities for personal development and meaningful contributions to your community.

For those who have emerged from addiction through the insights gained from self-study, personal determination, and proactive efforts, it's essential to engage in significant activities that involve using your experiences to help others.

Having successfully traversed the often tumultuous road of recovery, many feel a strong urge to give back. The insights and lessons you've learned from your journey are invaluable for others navigating similar paths. By telling your recovery story, you can provide hope, practical advice, and guidance to those still fighting the battle of addiction or just beginning their recovery. Taking on a mentoring or supportive role not only helps reinforce your own sobriety but also inspires others.

Let's explore a few key points that encapsulate the essence of this chapter:

1. Mentorship in Recovery

Mentorship serves as a meaningful way to channel your experiences into helping others. If you've navigated through addiction and recovery, you have the potential to offer profound support, encouragement, and advice. Mentoring enables you to connect deeply with others, sharing your experiences to help them face their fears and uncertainties.

Supporting Early Recovery: Those at the beginning of their recovery journey often feel confused and worried. Your personal experiences can bring them reassurance that they, too, can achieve recovery. Mentorship provides a welcoming space for them to ask questions and voice concerns, gaining comfort from someone who has faced similar hurdles.

<u>Providing Accountability</u>: Accountability is crucial during the recovery process. By stepping into a mentor role, you foster a sense of responsibility that can help others stay focused on their sobriety goals. Regular check-ins and open lines of

communication can help them remain accountable and reduce the risk of relapse.

2. Peer Support and Sponsorship

Many recovery programs highlight the significance of sponsorship and peer support. A good sponsor—someone with sustained sobriety—can guide others through their recovery process. As a sponsor, you play a key role in someone's journey by offering emotional support, providing recovery tools, and helping them navigate the ups and downs of staying sober.

<u>Sharing Insights</u>: Having experienced addiction personally, your practical advice can greatly resonate with others in recovery. By offering strategies for managing cravings, dealing with emotional challenges, and facing tricky social situations, you equip them to build a solid foundation for their sobriety.

Creating a Supportive Network: A major advantage of peer support is the sense of community it fosters. By integrating into someone's recovery network, you help create an environment where individuals feel safe, understood, and supported.

3. Volunteering in Recovery Communities

Many individuals find deep satisfaction in getting involved with recovery communities. Whether through leading support groups, organizing recovery-related events, or volunteering at rehabilitation centers, these actions provide meaningful opportunities to give back. Volunteering not only aids others in their recovery but also reaffirms your own commitment to staying sober.

Making an Impact: Volunteering allows you to directly change lives. By dedicating your time and energy to recovery initiatives, you help cultivate a supportive atmosphere that encourages healing and growth.

Reinforcing Your Own Recovery: Assisting others along their recovery journeys can enhance your sense of purpose and strengthen your commitment to sobriety. Witnessing the progress and success of those you help serves as a powerful reminder of your journey, motivating you to continue along your own path of recovery.

Chapter 7: How to Share Your Story and Inspire Change.

Your journey through recovery is a powerful opportunity to inspire change—not just for yourself but also for others and the broader community. By sharing your experiences, you can offer hope and motivation to those grappling with addiction. This openness can help dismantle the stigma often attached to addiction and recovery, promoting understanding and kindness. That said, when sharing your journey, it's vital to approach it with care, honesty, and authenticity to ensure your message resonates with those who hear it.

Here are some ways to effectively share your story:

1. Crafting Your Narrative

When you tell your recovery story, it's essential to create a narrative that's both engaging and relatable. Focus on significant moments that illustrate the obstacles you encountered, the pivotal choices that led you to seek help, and the valuable lessons you've learned along the way.

Embrace Honesty and Vulnerability: Authenticity is crucial. Be candid about your struggles, mistakes, and the vulnerabilities you faced. This openness helps others understand that recovery is not about perfection but about resilience and personal growth.

Highlight Your Growth and Transformation: It's important to not only acknowledge the struggles of addiction but also to share the positive transformations that have come from your recovery journey. Talk about the improvements in your life, such as rekindled relationships, better health, or a renewed sense of purpose.

<u>Provide Practical Advice</u>: In addition to sharing your story, consider offering practical strategies that have supported your sobriety. This could include tips for coping with cravings, mindfulness techniques, or ways to manage stress and emotional challenges.

2. Choosing the Right Platform

You have various avenues to share your experiences, ranging from personal conversations and support groups to public speaking and online platforms. Select the medium that best suits your comfort level and the audience you aim to reach.

Public Speaking: Sharing your story at recovery events, schools, or community organizations can be incredibly impactful. Public speaking gives you the chance to connect on a personal level and provide inspiration to those seeking hope.

Social Media and Blogging: Online platforms offer a way to share your recovery journey with a wider audience. Through blog posts, videos, or social media updates, you can reach people who may not have access to traditional recovery resources.

Writing and Publishing: If you enjoy writing, consider documenting your experiences in articles, books, or online forums. Written narratives can connect with a broader audience, providing a lasting resource for those on their own recovery paths.

3. Inspiring Advocacy and Social Change

Your personal narrative can also be a powerful tool for advocating broader social change. Addiction is frequently misunderstood and stigmatized, and by sharing your story publicly, you can help reshape the conversation around it. Advocate for improved access to treatment, more support for recovery programs, and education about the realities of addiction.

Breaking Down Stigma: Sharing your experiences can humanize the issue of addiction, helping to dismantle damaging stereotypes. When people hear firsthand accounts of recovery, they're more likely to cultivate empathy and support those still facing challenges.

Raising Awareness: Your story can also highlight the pressing need for addiction treatment and resources within your community. By raising your voice, you can inspire action and contribute to meaningful societal change.

In summary, your recovery journey is not just your own but it can be a beacon of hope and a catalyst for change. By sharing your story thoughtfully and authentically, you can inspire others, advocate for those in need, and promote a deeper understanding of addiction and recovery in society.

Chapter 8: Contributing to the Community/Society and Making a Positive Impact

Transforming your recovery journey into a source of empowerment also means seeking ways to make a positive impact in your community and society at large. Engaging in activities like volunteering, advocacy, and community outreach can instill a profound sense of purpose and fulfillment. These efforts contribute to creating a supportive environment where individuals feel valued and encouraged on their paths to recovery.

1. Volunteering in the Community

Volunteering is a fulfilling way to dedicate your time and talents to help others while making a significant contribution to your community. From organizing recovery-focused events to mentoring those in need, the opportunities to give back are numerous.

Community Outreach: Get involved in outreach programs aimed at supporting those at risk of addiction or in need of recovery assistance. This could take the form of workshops, educational events, or support group meetings designed to raise awareness and foster understanding of addiction and recovery.

Service-Oriented Initiatives: Many who are in recovery find deep satisfaction in engaging in service-oriented activities, such as organizing food drives, participating in charity events, or volunteering at local shelters. These acts of kindness not only uplift the community but also inspire others to contribute in meaningful ways.

2. Becoming an Advocate for Recovery

Advocacy offers a powerful platform to create lasting change within the community. Whether championing addiction treatment, mental health services, or reforms within the criminal justice system, using your voice to advocate for change can lead to significant, long-term impacts.

Partnering with Organizations: Team up with local or national recovery organizations to push for better access to treatment, resources, and support services. By collaborating with established groups, you can magnify your impact and help drive policy changes that support the recovery community.

Educating the Public: Take on the role of a public educator by sharing your insights and experiences at schools, workplaces, or community centers. Providing information on addiction, recovery, and mental health can help prevent future cases of addiction and foster a more supportive environment for those in recovery.

3. Creating a Lasting Legacy

Your journey of recovery is a remarkable testament to resilience, growth, and the incredible potential for change within all of us. By giving back to your community, supporting others, and advocating for positive change, you have the opportunity to build a legacy that extends beyond your personal experience. Inspire others to believe in their own capacity for healing and growth, and in doing so, contribute to a larger movement of hope and recovery within society.

Summary

In *Chapter 6: Turning Your Journey into Empowerment*,
This chapter emphasizes how your recovery journey can become a wellspring of strength, insight, and inspiration for those around you. By utilizing your experiences to mentor others, share your story, and give back to your community, you not only reinforce your own sobriety but also play a vital role in fostering healing and empowerment in others. It provides a guide for transforming personal struggles into opportunities that create a meaningful impact on the lives of those in need.

Acknowledgments

First of all with a praiseful heart, I really and thankfully appreciate the creator of the universe. I call him the being of beings, for giving me the inspiration to gather my experience, gospel and message, and put them to writing despite how long it took me, just for the world to benefit from the goodness of the message, information and education in this book.

Though I am a musician, I really had to write this book to make individuals who are vulnerable benefit and be changed for good.

I also appreciate most people who supported me in writing this wonderful book. I wish you all more than the good things you wish yourselves.

1. Personal Acknowledgments:

"To all my family members, whose true love and support carried me through my darkest hours. Without their belief in my ability to heal and grow, this book would not have been possible."

2. Professional Acknowledgments:

"To the competent team of recovery specialists who equipped me with the tools to reclaim my life. Your expertise and dedication inspired the core principles of this book."
Though, I am a musician but due to the love I have for writing and publishing of the truth and realities, I wrote this book. I thankfully appreciate all my aids who willingly encouraged me to write this book.

References

1. Books and Publications;

This subsection includes the titles of some key books and publications that have influenced my understanding of addiction, recovery, and self-improvement.
For further studies of all my readers who fine this book interesting, these below books are the key books that has influenced me;

Samuel C.A Adolphus (2024). *Understanding The Key Ideas Of Mastery. Amazon Kindle store.
- Smith, J. (2015). *The Science of Addiction: Understanding the Biology of Cravings and Recovery*. HarperCollins.

- Johnson, L. (2018). *Mindfulness in Recovery: How Meditation Helps Overcome Addiction*. Random House.

2. Academic Journals and Studies;

Citing peer-reviewed journals and studies is crucial to validate the scientific aspects of my work. This subsection includes research on the biological and psychological factors of addiction, the effectiveness of various recovery treatments, and the impact of mindfulness or therapy on long-term sobriety.

- *Miller, W. R., & Rollnick, S. (2013). "Motivational Interviewing in Addiction Treatment." *Journal of Substance Abuse Treatment*, 45(3), 345-356.*
- *Davis, R. A. (2020). "The Role of Neuroplasticity in Overcoming Addiction." *American Journal of Psychiatry*, 177(4), 256-264.*